Paleo Slow Cooker Soups & Stews
Delicious, Healthy, Nutritious and Gluten Free Recipes for the Entire Family

Table of Contents

About Paleolithic Eating

The Paleolithic diet, also known as the caveman diet, is a nutritional plan based on wild plant and animal based food sources. The dietary regiment mimics that of pre-agriculture hunter-gatherers. All humans consumed this diet in the Paleolithic era that began 2.5 million years ago and continued until 10,000 years ago when the development of agriculture introduced grain-based diets. The premise of Paleolithic eating is that humans are genetically adapted to the diet which every person consumed for a large portion of our history. It is composed of meats, seafood, fresh fruits and vegetables.

Practitioners of this diet should consume 60% animal foods and 40% plant foods. The diet excludes cereal grains, legumes, dairy, refined sugar, processed foods, salt and refined vegetable oils. The framework includes higher intake of protein, fiber, potassium, omega 6 and 3 polyunsaturated/ monounsaturated fats, alkaline foods, vitamins, minerals, antioxidants and plant phytochemicals. By eliminating foods, the diet lowers carbohydrate intake, glycemic index, and sodium. Consuming this diet has shown to reduce health problems such as weight gain, cardiovascular disease, diabetes, metabolic syndrome, and gastrointestinal tract diseases, to name a few. Going back to these basics, has shown promise to optimize health, reduce disease and maintain a healthy weight.

Overview

Within this book you will find recipes to help you follow the Paleolithic dietary guidelines. Life can be very busy and preparing meals, let alone meals that have specific rules for what can be included, can seem impossible. Every recipe in this book can be prepared in a slow cooker crock pot ahead of time for a stress free dinner time. The recipes are divided into 6 sections by the type of meat included in the recipe. The sections of recipes you will find are beef, chicken, vegetables, pork, lamb and then other meats. Enjoy these easy to prepare, nutritious and delicious Paleolithic slow cooker, gluten free, soups and stews.

Chapter 1: Beef Recipes

Beef and Mushroom Ragout

500g shin beef or chuck steak

1 large onion

150g mushrooms

150g diced bacon, low fat

100ml beef stock

100ml red wine

2 or 3 sprigs thyme

2 tablespoons flour, gluten-free plain flour or rice flour

1 can diced tomatoes

Olive oil

First you cut the beef into 2 -3 cm cubes and place it in a plastic bag with the flour and shake to coat the meat. Next chop the onion and slice the mushrooms. Oil a frying pan gently cook onions, chopped bacon and mushrooms until onions are soft. Place in a crock pot. Add a little extra oil and brown the meat a few pieces at a time then place in the crock pot. Deglaze the pan using the wine and pour it into the crock pot. Also, add the tomatoes, thyme, and stock. Cook on low for 9 hours and serve with rice and green salad.

Hearty Mushroom and Beef Stew

Olive oil for frying

2 large onions, thickly sliced

1 clove garlic, roughly chopped

500g diced steak, skirt or chuck

60 ml whisky

1 cup beef stock

Salt and pepper to taste

1 heaped teaspoon smoked paprika

1 teaspoon dried herbs de Provence

2 large mushrooms (like portabellas) chopped into large chunks

Corn flour mixed with water (if needed, about a teaspoon to a couple of teaspoons)

Start with the onions and garlic. Heat a large frying pan with olive oil on medium heat and add the onions, fry for 5 minutes and then add the garlic. Stir for another minute, then remove the onions and garlic with a slotted spoon and place into the slow cooker. Heat the pan to high and add more oil to cook the beef. Keep stirring with a wooden spoon. You want to sear the meat with a rich color quickly. After a few minutes this should have seared. Using a slotted spoon, remove and place in the slow cooker. There should be juices from the meat left behind in the pan. Add the whisky to the juices in the frying pan and stir for a two minutes. Lower the heat down to medium and add 1/2 of the stock. Pour the remaining 1/2 in the slow cooker. Stir the juices around in the frying pan and when bubbling carefully pour into the slow cooker. Next add the seasoning, paprika and herbs. Combine well and put the lid on. Cook for about 6 hours. About 2 hours before serving, place the mushrooms in the pot. Stir well and replace the lid. After about an hour and a half, check the consistency of the liquid. (Slow cookers tend to produce a lot of liquid). Try to get a runny to thick gravy consistency. Add corn flour mixed with water if you need to thicken it up, stir and cover. Serve in a deep bowl with bread on the side. Garnish with chopped flat leaf parsley.

"Yes Please" Beef and Bacon Stew

1 kg beef mince

230g bacon, diced

1 medium onion, diced

1 (400g) tin red kidney beans

1 (400g) tin tomato soup

1 tablespoon mustard

2 teaspoons Worcestershire sauce

You will start by lightly spraying the slow cooker with cooking spray. After that fry or microwave your bacon until lightly browned. Be sure to drain on paper towel. If using a frying pan discard bacon dripping. Next, in a heated skillet brown your onion and then add in beef. In a separate bowl combine bacon, beef and onion with the beans and soup. Transfer to slow cooker and cook on LOW for 7 to 9 hours. Stir in mustard and Worcestershire sauce before serving.

Beef Stew (Spicy)

750 grams beef meat (stew meat cubed)

5 cups beef stock

1 cup red wine

3 celery stalks, cut into 5cm pieces

3 garlic cloves

4 onions, chopped

1 tsp. salt

1 tsp. ground black pepper

1 tsp. ground cayenne pepper

810g can whole peeled tomatoes

4 carrots, sliced

1/2 tsp. chili flakes

1 tsp. oregano

1 tbsp. dry mustard (ground)

Mix together beef, stock, wine, tomatoes, carrots, celery, garlic and onions in your crock pot. Season with salt, pepper, cayenne, and chili flakes, oregano, and mustard. Cover and cook on low 10 to 12 hours. Then Enjoy!

Sweet Beef Stew

1 pound stew beef

1 tbsp. coconut oil

1 carrot

1 medium onion

1 tsp. cinnamon

1 cup beef broth

Heat coconut oil in a crock pot turned to high heat. (If oil is hard, allow it to melt and coat the bottom of the cooker.) Chop the carrot and onion into bite-size chunks and add to the crock pot. Next add stew beef chunks and beef broth. Let the combination cook on high heat for approximately 2.5-3 hours. Sprinkle cinnamon over the mixture and stir to combine. Turn the crock pot down to low until you are ready to eat.

Paleo Taco Soup

1 pound ground beef

1 red onion, chopped

4 garlic cloves, minced

1 tbsp. chili powder

1/4 tsp. garlic powder

1/4 tsp. onion powder

1/4 tsp. crushed red pepper flakes

1 /4 tsp. dried oregano

1/2 tsp. paprika

1 tsp. ground cumin

Dash of salt and pepper

2 cups chicken broth

1 4 oz. can of fire roasted green chilies

4 medium tomatoes, diced

1 cup salsa

Heat a large pan over medium heat until pan is hot, then add the ground beef and brown it using a colander. Then drain the fat from the meat (if desired) and add it to the crock pot. Combine all other ingredients into the crock pot and cook on low for 6-8 hours. Garnish the soup with sliced avocado or cilantro.

Okra Beef Stew

2 cups chopped okra

1 lb. beef stew meat, chopped

2 medium tomatoes, chopped

1/2 yellow onion, diced

2 carrots, thinly sliced

2 cups chicken broth

1/2 cup tomato sauce (any kind you have on hand)

2 tsp. paprika

2 tsp. garlic powder

1 tsp. black pepper

1 tsp. onion powder

1 tsp. cayenne pepper

1 tsp. dried oregano

1 tsp. dried thyme

1/4 cup sun dried tomatoes, chopped

Combine all the ingredients together except the sun dried tomatoes. Add them into the crock pot and stir well. Cook for 7 hours on low heat. Then divide stew between bowls and top each with sun dried tomatoes.

Beef Heart Chili Stew

1 cup of heavy beef broth

1 beef heart

2 strips of uncured bacon

1 yellow chopped onion

1 green bell pepper, chopped

4 cloves of garlic, minced

Splash of balsamic vinegar

1 can of fire-roasted tomatoes

1 can diced tomatoes

1/2 cup water

2 tbsp. chili powder

1 tbsp. paprika

1 tbsp. ground cumin

1/2 tsp. cocoa powder

1/2 tsp. cinnamon

Salt & pepper to taste

The first thing you need to do is clean your beef heart. It takes some time and a decent knife, and you must cut off all the hard fat as well as any connective tissue. You cut the heart into cubes and set aside for later. Then, in a large skillet cook until browned diced bacon over medium heat. Put the bacon in your crock pot and save the drippings. Turn the heat up and sear your beef heart in the bacon fat for a few minutes, until browned all over. You may need to add more bacon fat if your two strips don't render enough. Next add your onion, bell pepper, garlic, both cans of tomatoes, water, and all spices to your crock pot. Combine well. Next go back to your heated skillet and add just a splash of balsamic vinegar and scrape up any bits of bacon and beef heart. Add all the beef heart and all the flavor to your crock pot. Cook for 7-8 hours on low.

Moroccan Beef Stew

2 lbs. beef, cubed

5 tbsp. olive oil/butter

2 large onions diced

5 cloves of garlic minced

4 large carrots chopped

1 large sweet potato diced

1/2 cup raisins

1 cup strained tomatoes

1 inch piece of ginger, minced

1 tbsp. freshly ground black pepper or more to taste

1 tbsp. each ground cinnamon, turmeric, paprika

1 tsp. cayenne powder or more to taste

1/2 cup beef broth/stock

Juice of 1 lemon

2 cinnamon sticks

Salt to taste

Start with the spices, crush and mix them together and cover the meat and mix well. Let that sit. Heat half the oil/butter in a large pot and sauté the onions until browned over a low heat for 15 minutes. Next combine the garlic and ginger and continue browning another 5 minutes until the onions lightly caramelize then remove from heat and add to crock pot. Brown the meat in the remaining hot oil, in two batches then add that to the crock pot. Add the strained tomatoes and stock to the crock pot next and bring to a boil, scraping the bottom. Add the tomato liquid to the crock pot. Add all remaining ingredients and stir well.

Cook for 6-8 hours on the low heat setting (or high for 4 hours) checking and stirring occasionally.

Serve on cauliflower rice.

Beef and Butternut Squash Stew

2 lbs. grass fed stew beef

1 onion chopped

2 garlic cloves chopped

1 tbsp. rosemary

1 tbsp. thyme 2 tbsp. parsley

1/2 tsp. sea salt

1/2 tsp. pepper

1 cup red wine

1 butternut squash cubed

1/4 c sun dried tomatoes

4 cups organic beef broth

This is a very easy recipe. Just combine all the ingredients in the crock pot and cook for 6 hours. Sauté the onions and garlic in olive oil prior to putting them in the crock pot for added flavor.

Chili Stew

1 pound ground beef

1 can tomato sauce 28 oz.

2 c. beef broth

1/2 c. pureed pumpkin or carrots

2 c. mushrooms sliced

1 zucchini

1 onion

6 to 8 minced garlic cloves

2 tbsp. olive oil

3 tbsp. chili powder

1 tsp. garlic powder

Turn your crock pot to high and heat a large pan. Brown the beef, then add it to the crock pot. Next stir in the tomato puree, broth, pureed pumpkin or carrots, chili powder, and garlic powder to the crock pot. Drop the olive oil into the same pan the beef was browned in and sauté over medium heat until they have softened: onion, mushrooms, garlic, and zucchini. Mix into crock pot. Let cook on high for 1-2 hours then reduce too low for 4 hours.

Beef Shank Soup with Bok Choy

One pound beef shank with bone

4 cups of beef stock

4 cups of water

2 large carrots, peeled and sliced thick

2 to 4 stalks of celery, sliced thick

4 cloves of garlic

1 small to medium onion, quartered

1 large bunch of boy choy, base cut off

Salt and pepper to taste

In a crock pot, season your beef shank with salt and pepper. Next, lightly sear your beef shank in a skillet over high heat until it is browned on both sides. Put your seared beef shank, beef broth, water, carrots, celery, garlic, and onion into your crock pot. Place your bok choy on top of your fluid, floating on top of your liquid base. And cook on low for 4 hours.

Lime Beef Stew

1kg diced beef stew meat

1 peeled and diced sweet potato

2 chopped red onions

2 quartered limes

4 peeled and chopped cloves of garlic

2 tsp. of Spanish smoked paprika

3 lime leaves

2 bay leaves

1 tsp. ground cumin

1 tsp. ground coriander

1/2 tsp. ginger powder

1/2 tsp. salt and pepper to taste

1 can coconut milk

Combine all ingredients in a crock pot, mix well and cook on low for 7-8 hours. Serve hot with vegetables and enjoy.

Chapter 2: Chicken Recipes

Chicken and Tomato Stew

6 chicken breast fillets, cut into bite size chunks

1 onion, diced

2 cloves garlic, finely chopped

12 button mushrooms, sliced

2 carrots

3 sticks celery, diced

2 capsicums, diced

2 zucchini, diced

1 jar pasta sauce

Combine all ingredients in the slow cooker, cover and cook on low for 7 to 9 hours.

Manhattan Chicken Stew

1 lb. Skinless/Boneless Chicken Thighs (cut up into bite size pieces)

1 large can of diced tomatoes

1/2 cup chicken broth

1/2 cup dry red wine

1 large red onion minced

1 package of fresh sliced mushrooms

4-6 cloves of minced garlic

1 tsp. dried oregano

1 tsp. of dried basil

1 tsp. of kosher salt

1 tsp. of ground pepper

Combine all of the ingredients into your crock pot and cook for 6 hours on low heat. Stir occasionally. Add herbs and seasonings to your tastes. This is great with steamed veggies or as chowder.

Chicken Noodle Soup

3 cups chopped chicken, precooked

6 cups chicken stock

2 cups water

1 12 oz. bag broccoli slaw

Salt and pepper to taste

Combine all ingredients in the slow-cooker and let simmer on low for 5-6 hours or on high for 4 hours. Enjoy!

Chicken and Vegetable Stew

3-4 large chicken breasts

1 small head of cauliflower

2 cups of carrots

1 bunch of celery (about 6-8 stalks) chopped

2 zucchini chopped

2 onions diced

4 cloves garlic and 1 tablespoon olive oil minced

6 cups chicken broth

Salt and pepper to taste,

2 tbsp. curry

1/2 tbsp. cumin

1 1.2 tbsp. sweet paprika (not regular- sweet- can find at grocery store)

Combine your garlic and onion and put that and the olive oil in the crock pot on high heat. Chop up your cauliflower with all your other vegetables into bite size pieces. After that cut up your chicken into bite size pieces as well. Next, layer the ingredients into the crock pot and after each edition sprinkle some of your spices onto the mixture. Continue until all ingredients are in the crock pot. Lastly, pour your vegetable/chicken broth in. Cook on low for about 8 hours until the chicken is cooked thoroughly.

Chicken Enchilada Soup

500g boneless, skinless chicken breast halves

1 (400g) tin whole kernel corn, drain out juices

1 (400g) tin diced tomatoes with juice

130g diced green chilies

1 white onion, diced

1/4 cup fresh coriander, chopped

2 bay leaves

3 cloves garlic, minced

500 ml chicken stock

320g enchilada sauce

1 teaspoon ground cumin

1 teaspoon chili powder

1 teaspoon salt

1/4 teaspoon ground black pepper, to taste

Start by rinsing and patting dry the chicken breasts. Place them into the bottom of a slow cooker. Combine the corn, tomatoes, onion, coriander chicken stock, enchilada sauce, green chilies, bay leaves, garlic, cumin, chili powder, salt and black pepper. Cook for 6 hours on low heat. Remove the chicken to a large plate and shred the meat with two forks. Return the chicken to the slow cooker and continue cooking for 30 minutes to 1 hour.

Chicken Cacciatore Stew

1 whole chicken, cut up

2 large chopped onions

1 large can of diced tomatoes

2 large diced green peppers

1 teaspoon minced garlic

1/4 teaspoon red pepper flakes

2 Tablespoons dried Italian herb blend

Place cut up chicken in slow cooker and mix all other ingredients in a large bowl and combine well. Pour the mixture over the chicken in the crock pot. Cook for 6-8 hours on low until chicken is falling apart.

Smokey Chicken Stew

12 Boneless skinless chicken thighs (~1.5lbs), trim fat (chicken breasts optional)

1-2 Tbsp. Coconut oil

1 Onion, chopped pretty finely

2-3 Carrots, chopped

3 stalks Celery, chopped

1/2 container Mushrooms (optional)

4 cloves Garlic, minced

1/2 14oz can Tomato paste

1 Tbsp. dried Basil

28oz can Fire roasted, diced Tomatoes

8 oz. full fat Coconut milk or Coconut cream

Start by heating the coconut oil over medium heat and adding the onions, carrots, and celery. Cook for 5-10 minutes until they are partially softened and transfer to the crock pot. Then combine mushrooms, garlic, tomato paste, basil, and seasoning blend. Stir until all vegetables are coated in tomato paste. Then cut the chicken into smaller cubes (otherwise you will have to shred it later which can be tedious) Add to the crock pot and pour canned tomatoes and coconut milk over it all. Stir well and cook on high for 4 hours or until chicken and vegetables are cooked through. Then salt and pepper to taste and serve with another splash of coconut milk over the top to cool it down.

Crock Pot Chicken Spinach Soup

3 Chicken breasts

1 small bag spinach

2 large zucchini

1 medium onion

1 can tomatoes, diced

1/2 head cauliflower, chopped

2 cups water

2 teaspoons oregano

1/2 tablespoon thyme

Pinch ground red pepper

Start by cooking the chicken with 2 cups of water in a crock pot on low heat. Save the broth to add into the soup later. In large stock pot, cook the chopped onion and zucchini with a tablespoon of olive oil. Cook until the onions are translucent. Then add bag of spinach, oregano, thyme, ground red pepper, can of tomatoes to the onions. Cook until the spinach is softened. Then add the chicken broth that you saved from the crock pot. Add the chopped bite size cauliflower. Bring to boil, then lower heat to simmer for 10-15 min. Add salt and pepper to taste. And top with parmesan cheese (optional)

Chapter 3: Vegetable Recipes

Pumpkin Eggplant Stew

1 pumpkin butternut

2 c. eggplant

2 c. zucchini

1 packet okra

250g tomato (pureed)

1 c. onion chopped

1 tomato, chopped

1 carrot, slice

1/2 c. vegetable stock

1/3 c. raisins

1 garlic clove minced

1/2 tsp. cumin ground

1/2 tsp. turmeric ground

1/4 tsp. chili flakes

1/4 tsp. cinnamon ground

1/4 tsp. paprika

In a slow cooker you will mix the butternut pumpkin, zucchini, eggplant, okra, tomato puree, tomato, carrot, onion, garlic, stock and raisins. Mix in all seasonings. Then simply let cook low for 8 hours.

Cannelloni Beans and Cabbage Stew

1 small cabbage, thinly sliced

2 (400g) tins cannellini beans, drained

1 1/2 liters vegetable stock

1 bay leaf

4 tablespoons dry white wine

2 teaspoons rosemary, diced

2 teaspoons thyme, diced

1 onion, diced

Salt and ground black pepper to taste

This is very simple, combine all ingredients in the slow cooker and cook on high for 4 hours then enjoy!

Red Lentil and Pumpkin Curry Soup

1 1/2 kg pumpkin of your choice

1 leek

1 1/2 cups dried red lentils

1 1/4 liters vegetable stock

2 tablespoons curry

Start by chopping up the pumpkin. Then get your leek, peel off skin if desired, chop the leek then add to the slow cooker. Combine the dried red lentil beans with the pumpkin and mix very well. Add curry to the vegetable stock, mix and then add liquid mix to the vegetables. Mix thoroughly. Slow cook on low for 8 hours or on high for 4 hours. Then mash up with a potato masher. Serve with fresh crunchy bread if desired.

Corn Soup

2 (400g) tins whole kernel corn

3 cups (750ml) vegetable stock

1 large onion, diced

1 clove garlic, crushed

2 red chilies, finely diced

1 tablespoon chili powder

2 teaspoons salt

1 tablespoon parsley flakes

Black pepper to taste

1 3/4 cups (435ml) soy milk

60g dairy free margarine

1 lime, juiced

Start by combining corn, vegetable stock, onion, garlic, chilies, chili powder, salt, parsley and black pepper in a crock pot. Cover. Cook on low for 7 hours. Pour the vegetable mixture into a blender, filling the container no more than half way. Hold the lid of the blender with a folded kitchen towel and carefully start the blender using a few quick pulses before leaving it on to puree. Puree in batches until smooth and pour into a clean pot. You can also use a stick blender and puree the mixture in the cooking pot. Once you have pureed everything return it to the slow cooker. Stir in the soy milk and margarine to the mixture; cook on low for 1 hour more. Finish it off with some lime juice, and serve.

Paleo Pumpkin Leek Soup

2 pounds chopped and peeled pumpkin (canned puree)

2 Leeks washed and trimmed

1 garlic clove, crushed

2 tsp. olive oil

3 cups broth (chicken)

1 tsp. ginger

1 tsp. cumin

Sea Salt

Ground Pepper

Heat your pan to medium/medium high heat and combine olive oil, chopped leeks and garlic and cook until softened but not discolored. Season the leeks and garlic to taste with ginger and cumin. Cook one more minute with spices on. In the crock pot, combine spices on top of the pumpkin and pour broth over the top. Next add sea salt and pepper to taste, Cook on low for 4-6 hours, the last hour cook on high and serve hot.

*if using fresh pumpkin chunks, follow the directions below:

Season the leeks and garlic to taste with ginger and cumin. Cook one more minute with spices on. Put spices on top of pumpkin cubes and pour broth over the top. Add sea salt and pepper to taste Cover and cook LOW 6-8 Hours. I stirred mine occasionally to try to move the chunks so that they could cook as evenly as possible. At hour 6, break out the blender, pulse until it's the desired consistency then return to the crock pot and cook for 1 more hour on HIGH. Serve hot.

Roasted Red Pepper Sweet Potato Soup

2 huge sweet potatoes, peeled and cubed. This measures about 6 cups of cubes

One 14 ounce jar of roasted red peppers in water (drained)

One 14 ounce can of coconut milk. I use Trader Joe's light brand

1 cup of chicken stock

1 small yellow onion, large diced

2 cloves of garlic

1/2 tsp. black pepper

1/2 tsp. red pepper flakes

Combine in slow cooker on low for 4-6 hours. Use your immersion blender or if you don't have one, blend the ingredients with a food processor or blender. Do not blend it all the way, leave some chunks of potato in the mixture. Garnish it with red pepper flakes or chipotle flakes.

Butternut Squash Soup – 5 Slow Cooker Varieties

1 large butternut squash that you peel, seed, and cut in cubes. This should result in about 6 cups of squash. If you buy the precut veggies, you will likely need 2 packages. My large squash that weighed just over 3 pounds ended up yielding just over 6 cups of cubes.

1 can of coconut milk (14 ounces). I used Trader Joe's light coconut milk yet a "full fat" brand will result in a creamier end product.

2 cups of chicken stock. Don't feel guilty if you don't make your own, but you should!

1 granny smith apple that you peel, core, and cut into cubes

2 medium to large carrots, peeled and chopped into small pieces

That is the core recipe. Notice there are no seasoning or special flavors added. We'll get there next. For one large squash, you need a can of coconut milk, some chicken stock, an apple, and a couple of carrots to help make the color pop! With this basic recipe, you now have the basis for making an array of super easy and super awesome butternut squash soups! I wish there was more magic to it than this, yet it really is this easy. You will combine ingredients for 4 to 6 hours on your low setting. After that, you just need to stick your immersion blender in your crock pot for a minute and puree that goodness up. If you don't have an immersion blender. Well, I guess you'll just have to get your food processor or blender dirty. These recipes should yield you just over 2 quarts of soup.

Traditional Butternut Squash soup

1 large butternut squash (about 6 cups cubed)

1 can (14 ounces) coconut milk

2 cups of chicken stock

1 granny smith apple, peeled, cored, and cubed

2 carrots, peeled and chopped

1 tbsp. ground cinnamon

1 tbsp. ground nutmeg

Carrot Ginger Butternut Squash Soup

1 butternut squash

1- 14 oz. can coconut milk

1 cup chicken stock

6 carrots chopped

1" piece of ginger, grated

2 tsp. of ground cumin

2 tsp. of ground cinnamon

Apple Cider Spice Butternut Squash Soup

1 large butternut squash (about 6 cups cubed)

1 can (14 ounces) coconut milk

2 cups of apple cider

2 apples of your choice, peeled, cored, and cubed

1 carrot, peeled and chopped

1 tbsp. of ground cinnamon

1 tbsp. of ground nutmeg

Thai Curry Butternut Squash Soup

1 large butternut squash (about 6 cups cubed)

1 can (14 ounces) coconut milk

2 cups of chicken stock

2 carrots, peeled and chopped

2 heaping tbsp. of red curry paste

1 small red onion, chopped

1″ piece of ginger, grated

6 cloves of garlic, chopped

All recipes are to be cooked on low heat for 4 to 6 hours. Blend or puree when cooking is finished. That's it. An immersion blender is ideal for this. If you don't have one, let your mix cool before transferring it to a blender or food processor.

Garnish with anything from cinnamon and nutmeg, to curry powder, pumpkin seeds, and of course bacon.

African Sweet Potato Soup Recipe with Peanut Butter, Black-eyed Peas and Beans

1 tablespoon peanut oil

1 tablespoon red or green Thai Kitchen curry paste- hot or mild, to taste (start with less

If you prefer it mild)

1/2 teaspoon cinnamon

1 medium red onion, peeled, diced

4 cloves garlic, minced

1 large yellow bell pepper, cored, seeded, diced

1 jalapeño or other hot chili pepper, seeded, diced fine

1 14-oz. can black-eyed peas, rinsed, drained

1 14-oz. can white beans, rinsed, and drained

1 14-oz. can black beans, rinsed, and drained

1 quart light broth

1/2 cup 100% natural peanut butter melted in a half cup of boiled hot water (for one cup

Total)

1/2 teaspoon crushed hot red pepper flakes, or more, to taste

2 tablespoons chopped fresh cilantro

Juice from 1 big juicy lime

2-3 teaspoons organic brown sugar or raw agave nectar, to taste

Sea salt and black pepper, to taste

Heat the light olive oil in large soup pot then add the curry paste and cinnamon; stir for a minute to infuse the oil with spice. Next combine the onion, garlic, yellow pepper and jalapeño. Cook the veggies for 5-7 minutes, stirring until softened. Add the black-eyed peas, black and white beans, broth, melted peanut butter, cilantro and red pepper flakes. Bring the soup to a high simmer, cover, and lower the heat; keep simmering the soup and cook until the vegetables are tender, about 25 to 30 minutes. Stir in the lime juice and agave or brown sugar.. Season with sea salt and ground pepper to taste. Make sure it is warm throughout and season to taste.

Chapter 4: Pork Recipes

Stew with Pork

Virgin olive oil, as needed

6 cloves fresh garlic, chopped

1 large onion, sliced thin

4 medium carrots, chopped

4 cups thinly shredded green cabbage

Sea salt and freshly ground pepper, to taste

2 14-oz cans Muir Glen fire roasted tomatoes- diced

1 teaspoon rubbed sage

1 teaspoon each of: dried basil and parsley

Hot red pepper flakes, shake to taste

5-6 cups organic broth, as needed

8 oz. cubed cooked ham

Heat a skillet and add the chopped garlic, onion, carrots and cabbage. Season with salt and pepper. Combine the canned tomatoes, balsamic vinegar, sage, parsley, basil, and hot red pepper flakes and add to onion mixture. Next, pour in enough broth to cover the veggies completely. Cover and cook on high for 4 to 5 hours, until the carrots are fork-tender and the cabbage is soft. Add the cubed ham to warm through (if your ham is not precooked, add at the beginning). If you need to more liquid, you can add some extra broth. Cover and heat through for another twenty to thirty minutes until heated thoroughly. Taste test for seasoning additions. Add a pinch of brown sugar to balance the heat or tartness, if you need to. Salt and pepper to taste.

Spicy Crock Pot Chicken Curry Stew

750g chicken breast

1 onion sliced

1 clove garlic chopped

2 tablespoons medium curry powder

1 teaspoon turmeric

2 carrots peeled and sliced

1 fresh chili sliced

1 stalk lemongrass sliced

2 x 270g cans of light coconut milk

2 teaspoons cumin

1/2 teaspoon salt

1/2 teaspoon cinnamon

1 teaspoon pepper

1 tablespoon finely chopped/grated ginger

1 can water (use the coconut milk can)

2 kaffir lime leaves sliced (optional)

Cooking oil spray

Start by trimming your chicken and cut in 2 cm size chunks. In a non-stick pan brown the onion and using some oil spray. Next combine all the dry spices together and place all ingredients into the slow cooker. Mix well. Cook on low for 9 hours. You can add a Garnish of fresh coriander and serve with rice and chutney.

Bacon Jalapeno Butternut Squash Soup

1 large butternut squash (about 6 cups cubed)

1 can (14 ounces) coconut milk

1 cup of chicken stock

2 carrots, peeled and chopped

1 granny smith apple, peeled, cored, and cubed

2 jalapeno peppers, chopped. Remove the seeds if you desire less heat

6 ounces of crisped bacon, chopped

4 cloves of garlic, chopped

Cook on low heat for 4 to 6 hours. Blend or puree when cooking is finished. That's it. An immersion blender is ideal for this. If you don't have one, let your mix cool before transferring it to a blender or food processor.

Harvest Pork Soup

3 pound pork roast

2 medium sweet potatoes

1 medium rutabaga

1/2 acorn squash

1 apple

2 bay leaves

1 black pepper

1 tsp. dried onion

1/2 tsp. granulated garlic

1/2 tsp. cinnamon

Cut the pork roast, apple and vegetables into bite sized pieces. Combine in slow cooker with 2 cups of water and apple juice. Stir in the seasonings and set your slow cooker to low for 6 hours. Enjoy!

Chickpea and Ham Slow Cooker Soup

1 meaty ham bone

500 g uncooked chickpeas

5 carrots, chopped

Kernels from one ear of corn

1 pinch ground black pepper to taste

You will start by placing the chickpeas into a large container and cover with cool water to cover about 2 centimeters over the level of the chickpeas. Let the chickpeas soak for about 8 hours or overnight. After soaking, rinse the soaked beans and place them into a slow cooker. Place the ham bone in the slow cooker, and pour in enough water to cover the beans and ham bone by about 5cm again. Cook for 8 hours on the low setting. Skim any foam from the top of the soup, and remove the ham bone. Remove as much meat as possible from the ham bone, and return the meat to the slow cooker while discarding the bone. Stir in carrots, corn and black pepper to taste. Set the cooker on low and cook for 1 hour and then turn the heat up to high and cook 1 more hour.

German Stew

150 g cooked ham, cubed

2 cups dried brown lentils, rinsed and drained

3 cups (750ml) chicken stock

3 medium carrots, chopped

2 stalks celery, chopped

1 onion, chopped

1 teaspoon Worcestershire sauce

1 clove garlic, crushed

1/4 teaspoon freshly grated nutmeg

1/4 teaspoon caraway seed

1/2 teaspoon celery or traditional salt

Handful chopped fresh parsley

1/2 teaspoon ground black pepper

Start by putting the lentils in a 5 to 6 liter slow cooker. Next combine the chicken stock, carrots, celery, onion and ham. Season with Worcestershire sauce, caraway seed, nutmeg, garlic, choice of salt, parsley and pepper. Cover, and cook on low for 8 to 10 hours.

Chapter 5: Lamb Recipes

Irish Crock Pot Stew

1 1/2 pounds of lamb stew cubes (from the leg)

1/4 cup arrowroot

1 tsp. bacon grease

2 large onions, chopped

4-5 cloves of minced garlic

1 tsp. butter or ghee

3 carrots, peeled and roughly chopped

4 parsnips, peeled and diced

1 cup asparagus, chopped in 1/4-inch pieces

4 cups beef broth

1 cup water

Salt and pepper to taste

1 tsp. fresh thyme leaves (and more for optional garnish)

Start by placing the arrowroot in a gallon plastic bag. Add lamb cubes and shake until all of the meat is coated. In a Dutch oven (or heavy-bottomed pot), melt the bacon grease on medium-high heat. Add lamb cubes and brown on all the sides. Remove lamb from the pot and set aside. Add butter and onions to the Dutch oven and scrape the brown bits off of the bottom while cooking the onions over medium to add flavor. Next, add the broth and water, while continuing to scrape the cooked bits off of the bottom. Add lamb and bring to a boil. Reduce to a simmer and let cook for 45 minutes. Add carrots, parsnips, asparagus, thyme, salt and pepper. You can either cook for one hour or simmer until it's ready to serve then you can transfer to a crock pot. To let the flavors combine well and the vegetables to become tender, transfer the mixture to a crock pot and cook on low for 3 hours. Salt, pepper and season as needed. Then, transfer to soup bowls and add optional thyme leaves for garnish.

Slow Cooker Mexican Birria

3-4 lbs. lamb shoulder and neck bones (for stew)

4 guajillo chilies

3 ancho chilies

4 arbol chilies

1 can diced tomatoes

3 cups chicken stock

1 white onion, sliced

8 oz. white mushrooms, quartered

6 garlic cloves, minced

2 tbsp. vinegar

2 tsp. oregano

1 tsp. black pepper

1 tsp. salt

1 tsp. thyme

½ tsp. cinnamon

½ tsp. cumin

Chopped cilantro (garnish)

In a medium saucepan, bring about 3 cups of water to a boil. Also, heat a skillet over medium heat. Next, cut the stems off of the chilies and remove the seeds and veins. You want to toast the chilies in the skillet for 5 minutes. Then submerge the chilies in the boiling water and the stove off. Soak them for 20 minutes and the puree them with 2 cups of chicken stock, and can of tomatoes in a food processor or blender. Layer the bottom of your crock pot with the lamb meat and bones and cover with sliced onions, the chili puree, spices and garlic. Combine the remaining 1 cup of chicken stock and vinegar. Cook on low for 8-10 hours. In the last 3 hours, add the chopped mushrooms and stir the stew. Serve in a bowl over cauliflower, rice or accompanied by yucca fries. You can garnish with cilantro.

Autumn Lamb Stew

1 pound cubed lamb stew meat (if the meat came from a leg roast, save the leg bone to add to the stew)

1 tbsp. olive oil

2 tbsp. tomato paste

1 cup dry red wine

1 large carrot, sliced

1 large white sweet potato, peeled and diced

1 medium onion, diced

3 cloves garlic, minced

1 tsp. crushed dried rosemary

1 tsp. dried parsley

1 bay leaf

3 cups chicken or beef broth

1/2 cup pure pumpkin puree

Salt and pepper, to taste

Heat the oil in a large skillet over medium to medium-high heat and salt and pepper the meat and the bone, if using, then brown thoroughly. Remove the meat and bone from the pan and add to the crock of the slow cooker. Next you will add the tomato paste into the skillet and stir into the pan drippings to soften. Add the wine to deglaze the pan, stirring the wine and tomato paste together. Pour the mixture over the meat, then add the rest of the ingredients except the pumpkin. Cook on high heat for 6-8 hours on low heat for 8-10 hours. Before you serve, remove about 1/2 cup each of the broth and some of the potatoes, carrots, and onions. Add them to the base of a blender or a bowl and use an immersion blender. If you do not have one transfer soup to a blender or food processor. Blend the broth and vegetables. Add the pumpkin to the puree and blend again until well combined, you can add more broth if needed. Transfer the vegetable puree to the crock pot and stir. Cover and re-warm, about 20 min. Remove the bone and bay leaf and serve immediately.

To Die For Crock Pot Lamb Shank Stew

4 lamb shanks

1 sweet onion

1 tsp. kosher salt

Freshly ground black pepper

4 sprigs fresh thyme

1 tsp. olive oil

1 tsp. dried basil

10 whole, peeled garlic cloves, large ones cut in half

8 ounces mushrooms, brushed clean, large ones cut in half

1 tsp. Worcestershire Sauce

1/2 cup red wine

1/2 cup beef broth

1- 14 oz. can diced tomatoes

1 teaspoon dried oregano

Spread the onions on the bottom of a crock pot.   Heat a heavy skillet over medium-high heat and season and cover the shanks in worchestire sauce. Then add olive oil and put in the lamb shanks, flip until browned on all sides. Move the lamb shanks along with any browned bits from the skillet in the slow cooker crock pot and top with garlic cloves and mushrooms. In a bowl, combine the remaining liquids and spices and pour mixture into the crock pot. Cook on low for 6 to 8 hours and the lamb will become tender.

Chapter 6: Other Recipes

Manhattan clam chowder

3 (10.5 oz.) cans of chopped clams with the juice

6 cups original low sodium V8 juice or fresh vegetable juice

4 cups filtered water

1.5 – 2 lbs. yellow or sweet potatoes (depending on paleo diet)

1/2 large onion, chopped

3 – 4 stalks celery, chopped

1/4 to 1/3 cup dried or fresh parsley

1 vegetable or chicken bouillon cube, no salt added to reduce sodium

2 teaspoons black pepper or to taste

1 teaspoon white pepper

1 teaspoon dried oregano

1/4 teaspoon garlic powder

Sprinkle of sage

1 bay leaf

Salt to taste

Wash, peel, and chop your potatoes, and your onions and celery; Add them to your crock pot or large pot with 4 cups water, the bouillon cube, chopped clams with clam juice, parsley, black and white pepper, (salt), dried oregano, garlic powder, sage, and bay leaf; Stir, cover, and cook on a low for 6-8 hours or until potatoes are thoroughly cooked; When potatoes are cooked, remove the bay leaf and add in 6 cups low sodium V8   original vegetable juice or fresh vegetable juice (or plain tomato sauce, water, and salt); stir, and let simmer for 30 minutes before serving.

Southwest Turkey and Vegetable Crock pot Stew

2 cups cooked turkey shredded

5 cups turkey/chicken broth

1 medium zucchini, diced

1 small onion, diced

1 stalk celery, diced

1/2 green bell pepper, diced

1/2 red bell pepper, diced

2 cloves garlic, minced

1/4 cup prepared tomato salsa

1 tsp. chili powder

1 tsp. ground coriander

1 tsp. ground cumin

1 tsp. paprika

1/2 tsp. dried oregano

Salt and pepper, to taste

Combine all ingredients in your crock pot slow cooker and let cook for 6-8 hours on high or 8-10 hours on low.

.....or crushed as you prefer

1/4 cup balsamic vinegar

Turkey Leg Stew

1 turkey leg, skin removed

1/2 celeriac (celery root), peeled and chopped

1/2 swede, peeled and chopped

2 cups (500ml) chicken stock

Place the turkey, celeriac and swede into a slow cooker. Pour in chicken stock and cover with a lid. Cook on medium for 8 hours or low for 10 hours.

Bacon and Corn Chowder

1 kg smoked bacon bits -any off cuts are good and the smokier the better for fuller

Flavor

1 clove of garlic crushed

1 large onion

2 cans cream style corn

1 liter stock

Split peas

Salt and pepper to taste

Chop bacon pieces into reasonable size cubes...not too small as the size is what makes this so good. Chop onions...as chunky or as small as you like. Sauté the bacon and onion and garlic in a pan. Add to slow cooker with stock (if you like a thinner soup add more stock or water) add the soup mix/split peas. Leave to cook 4 hours minimum on high. Add the cream corn one hour before serving. Stir in well. Serve with crusty bread for a hearty filling meal